Vanessa Maia Rangel

The Body under Acupuncture

Vanessa Maia Rangel

The Body under Acupuncture

ScienciaScripts

Imprint

Cover image: www.ingimage.com

This book is a translation from the original published under ISBN 978-620-2-04142-3.

Publisher:
Sciencia Scripts
is a trademark of
Dodo Books Indian Ocean Ltd. and OmniScriptum S.R.L publishing group

120 High Road, East Finchley, London, N2 9ED, United Kingdom
Str. Armeneasca 28/1, office 1, Chisinau MD-2012, Republic of Moldova, Europe
Managing Directors: Ieva Konstantinova, Victoria Ursu
info@omniscriptum.com

Printed at: see last page
ISBN: 978-620-8-50402-1

The Body under Acupuncture.

Introduction:

The aim of this paper is to analyze what kind of body undergoes acupuncture therapy. For this study, I will compare two publications that indicate different ways of understanding the body undergoing acupuncture: the first, through the theories of Traditional Chinese Medicine and the second, through neuro-anatomo-functional Biomedical theories.

This comparison will be based on the approach to the historical construction of the body as an object of study by the Social Sciences and Public Health, highlighting the shift from understanding the body as a biological object to a body as a phenomenological object.

This approach will be exemplified by three clinical cases from the learning experience of the author/student of the Specialization Course in Acupuncture/Traditional Chinese Medicine and will result in the elaboration of the "remedied body" based on the theory of *"embodiment"*.

The aim of this paper is to discuss the possibility of the body model being fundamental to giving visibility to discourses about the efficacy of acupuncture, in other words, about knowledge in acupuncture, but which does not necessarily allow for an understanding of this practice itself.

This study is justified in that it aims to contribute to an understanding of the current field of acupuncture in Brazil and consequently the teaching of acupuncture, covering Traditional Chinese Medicine and Medical Acupuncture.

It aims to test the hypothesis that the incorporation of the acupuncture technique in the treatment of chronic pain based on neuro-anatomo-functional causality has contributed to the construction of acupuncture as knowledge legitimized by science, diverging from the understanding of the empirical therapeutic efficacy of acupuncture, based on the theories of Traditional Chinese Medicine, as well as the understanding of a salutogenic practice.

We'll start with an explanation of the problem of the body in acupuncture, not to define what it is, but to understand how it can be represented.

1 The Body: From Movement to Location.

According to Kuriyama (2000), the use of acupuncture points began around the first century BC. Prior to this period, manipulation of the body based on the principles of traditional Chinese medicine was carried out using the moxibustion technique, at identified sites on the patient's body, known as Mo. Mo would be the term to designate both the structure where the interference was made and the associated function, as well as covering the possibility of the union of Qi (energy) with Xue (blood).

In fact, Kuriyama (2000) states that Mo cannot be fully understood by modern Western language and discourse, since the Chinese understanding of Mo advocates an image, such as the vision of a phenomenon of nature (the example of a flowing river) and not the attempt to unite what has previously been separated, as is the case with the language and discourse of modern science and consequently Western discourse.

However, what is represented in Mo and can still be identified by Western discourse is the aspect of movement. In this way, even though it is not possible to understand Mo by identifying its parts, because there are no parts in MO, it is possible to understand what Mo represents. Mo represents movement, change, transformation, transmutation, the cycles of life, emotional dynamics, passing time, in other words, MO represents vital dynamics.

If this makes sense, then Kaptchuk (1973) and Campbell (2001) are wrong to describe the theories of traditional Chinese medicine as static. On the contrary, when the principles of Yin and Yang are evoked, one can understand the image of Mo in the body and its manipulation, both through moxibustion and acupuncture needling.

So, as opposed to defining the mechanisms through which needling causes benefit for the patient, the visualization of Mo in the body is equivalent to the intention represented in Mo. The intention to interfere with this vital dynamic.

If this explanation is sufficient for an acupuncture apprentice, they can continue practicing, without angrily questioning its causality, but be content with its effectiveness, with the benefits they see in their routine activity. In other words, with the therapeutic action/phenomenon, which therefore corresponds to the interference in the patient's vital dynamics.

If this explanation is not enough for the learner, or if the learner is questioned about this causality, they will have to turn to theories of the body that explain the phenomenon of their practice by clarifying its structure in detail. In other words, by the anatomopathological theory of this body, which highlights the diagnosis, defines the nosology and locates the therapeutic intervention.

2 Two Possibilities in the Same Circularity

In order to highlight these two possibilities for the acupuncture apprentice, we are going to present two divergent models of the body that fit into the phenomenological representation model, conceived by the theories of Traditional Chinese Medicine, and the Western Medical model, attributed to biomedical theories centered on neuro-anatomy-physiopathology.

To understand these two models, we will consider acupuncture minimally as a technique, which refers to the use of needles on localized and external points of the body. Acupuncture allows access to the inside of the body through acupuncture points, where the outside and inside of the body are treated. Therefore, acupuncture could be explained by the possibility of externalizing the human body, i.e. when its interior is accessible for treatment through external acupuncture points.

This circularity (Hacking, 1999) shows that the technique and theory of acupuncture are closely intertwined and cannot be understood separately. We can observe this phenomenon of acupuncture both from the explanatory model (Kleinman, 1988) of Traditional Chinese Medicine and from the Biomedical Model, as we will see later.

However, the difference that will be highlighted between the two models presented below is that the signs that the patient shows on the outside of their body will represent the "internal disease", according to the theory of Traditional Chinese Medicine, while the signs expressed by the patient (symptomatology) will require the search for an internal explanation of the body in Biomedicine.

3 The Externalized Body: Representations of the Body in Acupuncture from the Nei Ching.

Yin and Yang in the Segmental Division of the Body.

The wise respected the laws of nature, so their bodies were free from foreign diseases; they lost nothing of what they had received from nature and their spirit of life never ran out. The Tao was practiced by the wise and admired by the ignorant. Obedience to the laws of yin and yang meant life; disobedience meant death. The obedient would rule, while the disobedient would live in disorder and confusion. Everything that goes against harmony with nature is disobedience and amounts to rebellion against nature.

The human species should respect the following system: The yin and yang of man were designed so that on the outside there is yang and on the inside there is yin. The yin and yang of the body are designed so that the yang is at the back and the yin is inside the front.

The yin and yang of the organs were designed so that the dense organs are yin and the hollow viscera are yang. Thus, the liver, heart, gallbladder, lungs and kidneys are yin, while the gallbladder, small intestine, stomach and bladder are yang. One should also conceive of the rule of yin in yin and yang in yang, such as the back being the yang region and the front the yin region.

Everything is arranged so that yin and yang complement each other on the front and back, inside and outside as feminine and masculine elements, and so that they serve and react to each other in order to harmonize with the yin and yang of heaven. This is why it is said that yin is active inside and acts as the guardian of yang and yang is active outside and acts as the regulator of yin.

The pure and resplendent element of light, which is yang, manifests in the upper orifices while the turbid element of darkness, which is yin, manifests in the lower orifices. Yang, the resplendent element of life, is represented by the four extremities and originates in the pores while yin, the element of darkness, moves towards the viscera. Yang creates air and yin creates flavors.

Tastes regulated by yin emanate from the lower orifices and air, which is controlled by yang, emanates from the upper orifices. If yang is victorious there will be heat, if yin is victorious there will be cold, and cold harms the body while heat harms the spirit.

When the spirit is hit, severe pain follows and when the body is hit, swelling follows. When the yang is strongest, the body is hot, the pores are closed and people start panting, they become violent and rude and there is no perspiration at all. People become feverish, the gums dry out, the stomach becomes oppressed and people die of constipation.

When yang is stronger, people can endure winter, but they can't endure summer. When yin is strongest, the body is cold and perspiration appears regularly all over it. People clearly understand their fate, shiver with fear and freeze, their full stomach stops digesting and they die. When yin is strongest, people can endure summer, but they can't endure winter.

Thus, if yin and yang alternate, their victories vary, as do their illnesses. In order to ascertain whether yin or yang predominates, we need to know whether a soft, low-tension pulse predominates over a strong, jumping pulse. During a yang illness, yin predominates and during a yin illness, yang predominates.

Yin and Yang in the Representation of the Internal Signals of the Body.

It is said that in ancient times the ancient sages discussed the human body and listed each of the viscera and intestines separately. They talked about the origin of the blood vessels and the vascular system and said that there are six junctions at the points where the blood vessels and arteries meet. Following the course of each of the arteries are the 365 vital points for acupuncture. Each of these points has a place and a name.

They could also explain what these viscera looked like on the outside. The heart is the root of life and gives rise to the versatility of the spiritual faculties. The heart influences the face and fills the pulse with blood.

The lungs are the source of respiration and the dwelling place of animal spirits or lower souls. They influence body hair and have an effect on the skin.

The kidneys (testicles) bring to life what is dormant and closed, they are natural organs for accumulation and the place where secretions are stored. They influence the hair on the head and have an effect on the bones.

The liver causes maximum fatigue and is the dwelling place of the soul or spiritual part that ascends to heaven. It influences the nails and exerts an effect on the muscles, generating animal desires and vigor.

Thus, a person's color shows when the heart is in a splendid state. The heart dominates the kidneys. The lungs are related to the skin. The state of the hair and body shows when the lungs are vigorous and splendid. The lungs dominate the heart. The liver is related to the muscles. The state of the fingernails and toenails shows when the liver is vigorous. The liver is dominated by the lungs. The berry is related to the flesh. The color and appearance of the lips show when the stomach is vigorous and splendid. The berry gives rise to the lungs. The kidneys are related to the bones. The state of the hair on the head shows when the kidneys are vigorous. The berry dominates the kidneys.

What is produced by yin originates from the five tastes; the five organs that regulate the body are affected by the five tastes. When acidity exceeds the other tastes, the liver is affected, forced to produce excess saliva and the strength of the berry is reduced. If salt exceeds the other tastes, the large bones will become fatigued and the muscles and flesh will become deficient and the spirit discouraged. If sweet exceeds the other tastes, the heart's breathing will be asthmatic and full and the strength of the kidneys unbalanced. If the bitter exceeds the other flavors, the atmosphere of the berry will become dry and that of the stomach dense. If sour exceeds the other tastes, the muscles and pulse will become sluggish and vigor will suffer.

We can see that the internal body, organs and viscera are accessed from the outside of the body, through the acupuncture points and the body's external signals, reflecting the involvement of the internal organs.

In addition to the body's external signs, access to the wrist can show visceral involvement. The wrists can be small, large, slippery, rough, light or strong and represent the same characteristics as the viscera.

They can also be described by color, such as when the pulse looks red and there is a stubborn cough, the observer can tell that there is air accumulated in the heart. When the pulse looks white and there is a slight cough, the observer may suspect that there is air accumulated in the thorax causing shortness of breath.

When the pulse has a green appearance, and can be compressed for a long time, the observer may suspect that there is air accumulated in the heart that is going down to the limbs and flanks because it has affected the liver, causing pain in the feet and head.

When the pulse has a yellow appearance, becomes large and slow and there is air accumulated in the berry, the observer may suspect that there is uncomfortable gas. When the pulse has a black appearance, the upper pulse is strong and large, the observer may suspect air accumulated in the small intestine, which is the yin region.

Yin and Yang in the External Signs of Death in the Body.

The sages discussed the importance of recognizing death through the signs shown in the body. Thus, when the pupil of the eye doesn't turn and remains stationary upwards, in the wrong direction, the color of the eyes is white and convulsions occur, there is involvement of the greater yang. Life is interrupted, sweats appear and then run out.

When the hundred joints relax completely, the eyes clench shut and stop working, the body's connections break, the ears deafen, the skin turns green and then white, the lesser yang is affected and death ensues.

When the face turns black, the teeth protrude forward and become filthy, the belly swells and closes and circulation ceases from top to bottom, there is involvement of the lesser yin with death.

When the belly swells, the patient can't breathe, followed by vomiting and the face turns red and then black, there is involvement of the greater yin and the skin and hair emit a sensation of dryness and heat when death comes.

When the tongue twists and becomes spongy and porous and shrinks against the upper gums, there is internal heat in the throat and disturbances in the heart, there is an impairment of absolute yin and death ensues.

It can be said that those who wish to know the inside of the body should examine the pulse and thus have the basis for diagnosis. Those who want to know the outside of the body observe death and birth. The pulse and the five colors are the most important means of diagnosis.

An example of the above statement is when the wrists of the arms indicate the state of the short ribs. The outer wrist of the arm denotes the state of the kidneys. The left outer arm pulse indicates the state of the liver, while the left inner pulse indicates the state of the diaphragm.

The right external pulse indicates the state of the stomach and the right internal pulse indicates the chest. The upper right external pulse indicates what is happening inside the thorax, while the upper left external pulse indicates the state of the heart. This is because anyone who knows how to listen to the pulse knows that when it is thin, slow and brief there is an excess of yang and when it is slippery, like pebbles rolling in a bowl, there is an excess of yin.

The Life Force, Disease and the Signs of the Body.

Treating and curing illness means examining the body, the circulation, the brightness or wetness of the skin and the pulse, to check whether it is robust or decaying and whether the illness is recent. When the body's vital forms are in mutual harmony, it means that healing is possible. When skin color and moisture are excessive, the disease can easily take hold. When the pulse is in accordance with the four stations, it means that the disease can be cured. When the pulse is weak and slippery, it is influenced by the vital forms of the stomach and this means that the disease can be cured if the appropriate season is chosen.

When the body's vital forms are in disagreement, the disease is said to be difficult to cure. When the skin is fresh, but not lustrous, it means that it is difficult to stop the disease. When the pulse is full and vigorous, it means that the disease has become increasingly serious. When the pulse is at odds with the four seasons, the disease is incurable.

Thus, the body is considered to contain what is subtle and tiny and is blamed for its ailments, for the discovery of which it is investigated.

By examining and pondering their conduct, a lot becomes apparent: the body, the physical appearance and the acupuncture treatment. The spirit, however, cannot be heard with the ear. The eye must be bright with perception and the heart must be open and attentive for the spirit to reveal itself. cannot be expressed through the mouth; only the heart can express everything that can be observed.

4 The Neurological Body: Representations of the Body in Medical Acupuncture

Campbel (2001) begins the third chapter of his book entitled "Acupuncture in practice: beyond points and meridians" by stating that modern acupuncture, also called medical acupuncture, differs from traditional acupuncture in that it employs the usual methodology of Western medical diagnosis, including complementary examinations. It does not use the tongue and pulse examination of traditional acupuncture and can be explained by the principles of anatomy, physiology and pathology, and therefore by the principles of medical science.

For the author, one of the benefits of this acupuncture model would be to be able to explain how acupuncture treats its patients, although he admits that this knowledge is directed only at the phenomenon of pain and not at other ailments, which are treated by acupuncturists.

The scientific argument is maintained when Campbell informs us that we need to wait for new discoveries about the organization of the central nervous system to understand, for example, why a patient can feel, during an acupuncture session, an irradiation of sensations that does not correspond to the known nerve pathways.

For Campbell, the difference between the two possibilities of acupuncture is clearer in the discourses of the groups trained in the traditional model and the modern model than in the consistent differences in practice, since surprisingly for the author, both are effective.

But what are these discourses that differ so much between groups of acupuncturists?

We can see that the discourse to which Campbell refers can be understood as a specific model of the body used by acupuncturists, who identify with the Biomedical model and which differs from the model already presented in Nei

Ching by Traditional Chinese Medicine.

This body model is defined by a neurosensitive surface, by the transmission of electrical and neurohormonal impulses through well-defined nerve pathways and by the translation of these stimuli into specific and differentiated parts of the hierarchically superior nervous tissue, therefore, it is a neurological body.

From this circumscription, the neurological body of medical acupuncture explains the effectiveness or ineffectiveness of the technique used in it by the same neurochemical principles, as in the case of explaining the effectiveness of acupuncture in cases of pain by the secretion of serotonin, endorphins and dopamines or its ineffectiveness in 20% of the population, attributed to the increased secretion of cholecystokinin in the central nervous system.

The explanation that we could attribute to the symbolic efficacy of the therapeutic phenomenon (Levi-Strauss, 1976) is also captured by medical science, when Campbell cites an earlier work of his, in which he states that the placebo effect must ultimately be a neurophysiological phenomenon.

Although he considers the differentiated situation of acupuncture as a therapy that intervenes in the patient's body through needles inserted manually by the acupuncturist and the possibility of this interpersonal interaction being beneficial in some way, the author does not elaborate on any possibilities outside the boundaries of neuro-anatomo-functional theory.

5 The Coincidences of the Externalized Body with the Neurological Body.

Campbell reports that when Western doctors began to take acupuncture seriously in the 1970s and 1980s, they noticed a similarity between certain acupuncture points called ashi and the newly discovered triggers points. Although they report that trigger points are not yet fully understood by Western medicine, they can be defined by painful areas, usually in muscle tissue from where pain radiates to distant areas of the body.

But it's not just the similarity in the understanding of what a traditional acupuncture point and a trigger point would be, but the possibility of locating the structures of the nervous system on the surface of the body.

The example of neurofunctional localization by pain was even used by Felix Mann (2000) who proposed a revision of the use of acupuncture points from traditional Chinese medicine by points located on anatomical structures determined by Western medicine to coincide with the localization of pain, as in the case of the replacement of point 20 on the gallbladder with the new trapezium point.

Although impressed by the coincidences in the two very different ways of understanding the body, Campbell states that not all theories about neuro-anatomical localization should be seen as legitimate causes of pain. An example of this appears in his critique of the so-called "piriformis syndrome", where he disagrees that it is the piriformis muscle that presses on the sciatic nerve, and that this painful syndrome may correspond to the existence of trigger points without the involvement of the nerve.

Campbell's argument shows that there is a suspicion that other anatomical possibilities may be responsible for the causality of the patient's gluteal pain, but there is no questioning of the structural causality itself.

So what is the coincidence between the externalized body and the neurological body? To answer this question, we'll turn to an aspect of Mary

Douglas' theory of the body (1970).

Douglas argues that the body symbolizes society in its structure, organization and beliefs. On the other hand, society also symbolizes the body through certain boundaries, in other words, society affirms places and positions of passage between what it considers the natural body and the social body. These boundaries, which can be exemplified by the anatomical structures of the body or the ways in which the body reacts to its environment, are regulated by society, or rather, by the different forms of knowledge that society constructs to regulate these boundaries.

It is important to make it clear that Douglas' theory (1970) does not deal with acupuncture, but we can use it to understand that the management of acupuncture points, as boundaries of anatomical structure or as boundaries of social relations, can represent different types of knowledge made available by acupuncturists to give intelligibility to the management of this body, at the same time as they constitute this body based on this knowledge.

The work of Douglas (1970) shows that the type and degree of care that society, through specific groups, exercises over the body reflects the concerns and anxieties of society or these social groups, which are made available in the body. Thus, the power relations of society and certain social groups will be available in the different ways in which this body is managed, which can be understood in the form of care, control, empowerment, etc.

As far as this work is concerned, Douglas' theory (1970) can clarify that the different ways in which the body is handled, based on care provided by the premises of Traditional Chinese Medicine and Acupuncture Medicine, may be representing the different knowledge/powers made available in the body, constructing the boundaries of intelligibility of this body for these different social groups.

We are now going to look at examples of acupuncture practice in order to make visible the construction of the boundaries between these two possible models of the body.

6 The Acupuncture Apprentice and the use of the two Body Models.

It was a first-time consultation. The patient had been referred by a neurologist with a diagnosis of chronic atypical facial pain. She reported having bilateral glaucoma 20 years ago, with a thrombosis in her right eye, when the pain began to be excruciating and unbearable. He had undergone various treatments, but the pain had not improved. It was decided to remove the eyeball due to the amaurosis and in an attempt to resolve the pain. After the removal of her right eye, the patient developed a strange sensation in her face, from the nose upwards, which was chronic but varied in intensity and radiated to the top and back of her head. This feeling of strangeness was diagnosed by the neurologist as atypical facial pain, and due to the lack of response to the prescribed medication: gabapentin 900 mg/day, nortriptyline 25 mg/day and sertraline 50 mg/day, she was referred to the acupuncture service. The patient also had a history of sadness and frustration due to the many cases of alcoholism in her family, a situation which contributed to the death of her only son.

Examination of the tongue showed slight redness, thinning and absence of a coating. Pulse examination showed deficient pulses on the left.

During the consultation, the acupuncturist tried to identify the pattern of disharmony presented by the patient. The pattern corresponded to the wind element, due to the instability, the upward movement of the head and the opening of the pathology in the eyes.

At the same time, the acupuncturist wondered if, during the extraction of the right eye, there had been any neural damage that could explain the patient's atypical facial pain or if it was a phantom pain. The acupuncturist asked the patient to bring all the most recent imaging tests, including a CT scan of the skull.

It was observed that the two body models were used to make a reasoning about the patient's pathology. While the traditional Chinese medicine model explained the body's interaction with the environment through a movement called wind, the biomedical model located the damage in the body, in the structure of the nervous system, which corresponded to the part of the face in the patient's body.

When choosing the initial therapy for the patient's first acupuncture session, the acupuncturist pointed out a few points that she called harmonizers, with an emphasis on the facial region and on trying to balance the deficiency and the movement of the wind. The acupuncturist agreed to closely monitor the patient's progress in terms of her symptoms, so that the therapy could follow the flow of the pathology, which would imply changing or not changing the acupuncture points.

It was noted that, despite the consideration of neuro-anatomical-functional causality, the acupuncturist opted, in the first session, for an approach more in line with the body model of traditional Chinese medicine, with therapy oriented towards the movement of pathology, understanding the acupuncture points as frontiers of openness and exchange between the body and the external environment.

Another example, also referring to a first-time consultation, was with a middle-aged patient who was referred to the acupuncture service for a complaint of chronic low back pain. During the anamnesis, the student investigated the patient's pain in detail, asking about the precise location, the intensity of the pain, its duration, the possibility of irradiation, the frequency, the association with movement and rest, as well as with changes in temperature. The student spent around 20 minutes assessing the pain. When she turned to the supervising acupuncturist, she was surprised to hear: "Forget the pain!". The student was confused. Throughout the patient's treatment, emotional aspects linked to anger at her lifestyle and limitations emerged as the main focus of her discomfort, a focus that was treated by the systemic approach of acupuncture, with an improvement in the patient's well-being, who in subsequent sessions no longer reported pain. She no longer remembered her main complaint. Symptoms other than pain were also addressed as they arose during the patient's follow-up.

In this case, the localization and specificity of the patient's pain were not addressed, but rather the emotional aspects related to it. The central emotion of the discourse, related to the examination of the patient's pulse, also mediated other aspects of her life and relationships, specifically with her work. The acupuncture points were again used as possible mediating boundaries between the suffering represented in her body and the incorporated aspects of her environment and life history.

These two examples of outpatient acupuncture practice show a tendency on the part of the acupuncturist to use knowledge based on the premises of Traditional Chinese Medicine, where the body can be understood as a relational body, in other words, where the management of acupuncture points seems to be done with the intention of mediating a process of suffering of the patient, represented in their body. But how can we understand the use of Biomedical knowledge mixed with Traditional Chinese Medicine knowledge?

To do this, we will look at the importance of scientific rationality in the Western world and in medicine in particular.

7 Representations of the body based on acupuncture paradigms

Santos (2005) states that the model of rationality that presides over modern science was formed from the scientific revolution of the 16th century, first developed in the natural sciences and then, in the 20th century, extended to the social sciences to form a global model. For this author, this is a totalitarian model in that it denies the rational character of all other forms of knowledge that are not guided by its epistemological principles and methodological rules.

Santos (2005) emphatically states that what characterizes this modern science and the global model associated with it is the systematic distrust of the evidence of our immediate experience, which is considered illusory. This is because this global model delimits knowledge that is intended to be utilitarian and functional, recognizing less the ability to deeply understand reality than the ability to dominate and transform it.

With its scientific rigor, it quantifies, disqualifies and objectifies phenomena, objectifies and degrades them, and by characterizing phenomena, it caricatures them.

On the other hand, Santos (2005) makes it clear that scientists themselves have questioned their paradigm, establishing that modern science is not the only possible explanation of reality, but rather a privileged form of knowledge based on the prediction and control of phenomena. As a value judgment, the scientific explanation of phenomena is the self-justification of science as the central phenomenon of our contemporaneity.

From a critical perspective of this scientific reason, Foucault (1997) is concerned with asking how a phenomenon happens. It is clear that the important thing is not to look for the transformations that a certain phenomenon or object has undergone, but to make it problematic and therefore historical. The author points to the importance of scientific knowledge/power in the construction of the body and its control, along the lines of laboratory control where scientific knowledge is created.

Kruse (2004) informs us that the analysis of the body runs throughout Foucault's work, valuing its positivity, because for Foucault it is not important to look for the body, but for the practices, experiences and relationships that strengthen or weaken it in each circumstance. In this way, in trying to pursue the conditions of possibility for the emergence of the ways of seeing and describing the body that we know today, we turn to anatomy and its insertion and organization in modernity, in order to understand the historicity of this way of knowing.

In his article on the historicity of the body, Flores-Pereira (2010) describes how the philosopher Rene Descartes (1989) is an important historical reference for the process of constructing a representation of the body that, in a more or less stable way, accompanies people in modern Western societies.

By constructing the statement "I think, therefore I am", which is considered to be the foundation from which the author builds his philosophy, Descartes proposes the separation of the person into two parts: the body and the mind. This process of dichotomizing the human person has two important consequences: the attribution of different social values to the body and the mind, as well as a gradual process of objectification of the human body.

The author informs us that in relation to the first consequence, we can see that it is the mind that the author attaches the greatest value to, since it represents thought and rationality which, in turn, would be distinctive characteristics of what it means to be a human being.

The body, on the other hand, comes to be seen as a different material from the person who "owns" it and is therefore given the meaning of something less valuable. This is exactly where the second consequence of the process of separating the human person comes in, namely the idea that the body is an object - different material, something that is "owned" - available for exploitative action by people.

The ability to intervene in the body in order to adapt it to the determinations of the environment in which it lives is then discovered and encouraged. In this context, the human body comes to be studied through a modern lens, that is, as an object that is distanced from the person (who is the mind, rationality) and which must be studied from its parts. A practical consequence of this process of objectifying the human body is that one area of science is assigned the main responsibility for studying it, in this case the medical sciences.

Flores-Pereira (2010) analyzes that the body, for this area of knowledge, is analyzed as an exclusively anatomical and biological object, an organism structured and ordered by organs and systems that perform defined functions and whose knowledge is a consequence of the integrated activities of, for example, anatomy, histology and radiology. The body is not a person, but an object at the service of people.

But so far we have tried to understand the knowledge about the body that defines it as a possible externalized body and a neurological body, based on the rationalities of Traditional Chinese Medicine and Biomedicine, respectively. We will now turn to the history of the practice of Western Medicine, in an attempt to clarify why the acupuncturist mixes these two knowledges in the management of the body of the suffering patient undergoing acupuncture.

8 The Practice of Western Acupuncture: The Importance of Therapeutics

"What have I found here? Pain, calm and peace. You have magic hands" (a patient's words at the time of needling).

If we have already managed to elucidate the complexity of the current direction of knowledge about acupuncture, we will now try to address its practice. We will use Sayd's (1998) historical approach to Western Medical Rationality to understand when the scientific theories justifying the neurological body emerged and developed, and the possible consequences of this style of thinking for acupuncture as a medical practice.

According to the author, in her studies on the history of medicine, the doctor is first and foremost a therapist who fulfills a promise: to serve.
Therapeutics - the art of healing, the obligation to treat the sick - deals with the human condition, with the fear of death and suffering.

The beginnings of Western medicine can be found in Greece, where, for the first time, illness and death lost their magical and punitive character. Healing practices were separated from magic.
At this time, the Greek deities reflected the various facets of medicine: Apollo - is the deity who presides over the arts and who teaches the medical arts to mankind. Asclepius - is the son of Apollo and possesses the art of remedying and relieving pain. Hygeia - is the daughter of Asclepius and represents health and vital strength. Panacea - is the daughter of Asclepius and represents the healing power of herbs.

Thus, therapeutics is a way of relating man to nature, with healing being the return to health. In Greek medicine, man's relationship with Hygeia is clearer than with Panacea. The very term "therapeutica" derives from the Greek verb meaning to serve, to provide assistance, meaning that the Greek doctor only cured what nature could cure. The doctor intervenes as a regulator in the relationship between man and the environment.

In this way, Higeia is a form of relationship with nature where preservation and maintenance are privileged. Panacea, on the other hand, is the possibility of healing through transmutation, through change, through forces external to man. This is why the remedy differs from food and diet.

It is important to understand that the search for a remedy in the environment is a human activity as old as the search for food. In Greek medicine, the remedy was understood as the nectar of Olympus, the possibility of overcoming death. In the 5th century, the first empirical knowledge of the human body and its phenomena (PHYSIS) appeared. It was during this process that illness became secularized and became part of the natural world of human life.

Greek medicine, by including human nature in PHYSIS, became suspicious of the Panacea. Thus, health can only arise from the individual himself. Associated with virtue, it was opposed to the use of medicine, as it was seen as an artificial cure. During the Hellenistic period, Alexandrian physicians took a greater interest in medicine. The oriental influences brought by Alexander the Great included new drugs that were soon incorporated by the Greeks and later the Romans.

But the definitive shaper of Western therapeutics at the time was Galen, who practiced medicine in Rome as a gladiator's doctor. Galen claimed to be a follower of Hippocrates, he used the notion of illness as an imbalance or plethora of the humors, and for him, the remedy was an altering element of PHYSIS. He discovered a remedy that would become a kind of Panacea - a remedy that would work for everything. His proposal was to administer a polypharmacy, so that the body would be able to seek out the substance that was most appropriate for its condition and the rest would be eliminated.

Galen's medicine remained active and undisputed throughout the Middle Ages, but due to religious influences during the supremacy of the Catholic Church, the healing power of nature or Hygiene was shifted towards the vision of healing through magic and the supernatural. In the Christian view, life on earth has no value and the reflection becomes one of finding the truth in divine criteria. Thus, the great criterion of truth in medicine, philosophy and all areas of knowledge becomes the weight of tradition and religious dogma.

As early as the Renaissance, the search for the new shifted from theocentrism to humanism. It was the time of the first formulations of what would become our science, with a curious and avid empiricism. Renaissance man then separated himself from religious dogma and asserted his creative power in the world, setting himself up as the master of nature.

While in Galenic medicine, which dominated the West from the 1st to the 19th centuries, everyone practiced the use of cathartics, because all the theories justified the need for elimination, in the Renaissance, healing came from something outside man, something that transformed and purified him.

The birth of modern medicine with the arrival of the Enlightenment considered that reality was rational, and that this rational world was clear, univocal, through observation via the senses. Understanding and knowledge came from observation. Thus, illness, the fruit of magic, lost its status and became a natural event.

Classificatory medicine was created, where each disease was seen as having its own existence. The search for a cure could only be based on rational proposals, derived from the observation and classification of diseases and the elements of nature that could serve as remedies.

In terms of medical therapy, two perspectives marked the 18th century: mechanism and vitalism. For Stahl - a vitalist - man is an indivisible whole. Stahl is a Hippocrat and his medicine is expectant. For Hoffmann - a mechanist - the organism is governed by the movements of the humors and the body is understood as a hydraulic machine. Although they were two different currents, both Stahl and Hoffmann believed that the best way to achieve health was through self-care, observing what was good or harmful for the body itself, so as to avoid going to the doctor as much as possible.

This idea of recommending listening to one's own nature and avoiding going to the doctor means that, since the Renaissance, the doctor has suffered a growing crisis of prestige as theories and therapeutic practices have become increasingly prolix and disparate.

At the end of the 18th century, medicine began to change. Hospitals, which until then had served as dispensaries for the poor, were transformed into treatment centers. Classification medicine will disappear and give way to the contemporary method. - The notion of human tissue and histology created by Bichat (1771 - 1801) allowed for the correlation of the clinic with anatomopathology.

The new medicine is therefore a knowledge that breaks with the classical episteme that thinks of man in relation to nature and inaugurates the contemporary episteme, characterized by the possibility of thinking of man as object of study of himself. With this conviction, doctors were able to abandon traditional medicines while searching for therapies that were consistent with the new approach to the world: that safe and controllable knowledge of the body was possible. This attitude towards traditional medicines and the theoretical systems that supported them, as well as the refusal or abandonment of their application, are considered to have marked the birth of anatomo-clinical medicine.

However, contemporary medicine was born without a therapeutic proposal of its own, just like the classificatory medicine of the species that preceded it, being more a method of approaching disease than an idea, a theory or a method of treatment and cure. Bichat's revolution brought a new understanding of the disease process through the association of symptoms with injury, but did not allow for any therapeutic inferences, i.e. the morphological aspects related to the process of falling ill and dying do not account for the dynamics of life and therefore do not allow for the thought of healing processes.

At this time, vital dynamics were obscure, but it was physiology, developed step by step with contemporary chemistry, that led to the elaboration of the first therapeutic systems free from Galen's theories of humors and the last vestiges of alchemy. The first system organized on this basis was Broussais (1772-1838), a doctor at the Paris Military Hospital, who imposed a system of treatment whose theoretical basis was entirely new: that disease was the result of a reaction by the organism to the environment, causing a process of inflammation and the organism's ability to react to stimuli or aggressions from that environment.

Throughout the 19th century, Claude Bernard (1813 - 1878) continued his work, refining the experimental method and using animals in observations and testing hypotheses, definitively consolidating physiology as a rigorous and independent discipline. But at this time, the new knowledge about the body and disease and even the first products of pharmacology did little to change the arbitrariness of doctors' therapeutic practices. Although the promising indications of physiology and pathophysiology had overcome Galen's humoralism once and for all, it was not able to create a new therapeutic method, and there were no significant novelties in medical practice derived from the new sciences.

Thus, from the 18th century onwards and much more strongly in the 19th century, the discrediting of medicine was evident in the abundance of publications entitled "medicine without a doctor", where there was no discrediting of medical science, but against doctors. This was because the novelties in therapeutics were infinitesimal compared to other knowledge about the life sciences.

The eighties of the 19th century saw a transition. The decade begins and all discourses can be called vitalist; the fight against therapeutic skepticism is experienced as militancy. Treatment should be eminently functional and patient-centered, with formulas prescribed for each patient.

In the meantime, the postulates of Koch (1843 - 1910) convinced the last non-believers in microbiology. Other bacteria were discovered and Pasteur (1822 - 1895) dramatically saved a young man with anti-rabies serum in 1885. In 1889, Behring (1854 - 1917) managed to control diphtheria with anti-diphtheria serum and so microbiology became an indisputable part of medicine: instead of being just another item for etiological discussion, it became involved in the development of the disease. The acceptance of the existence of bacteria as disease-causing microorganisms is followed by a series of changes, as they make up a picture, from which a new context and a new role for therapeutics finally emerge.

It is important to note a change in tone, regardless of whether or not there is a "more correct" medical conception. Until 1890, vitalism was the most widely used source of argumentation for all the disciplines that make up medicine, especially for therapeutic discussion. From then on, the mechanistic explanation gained momentum, the disease became an autonomous being, because the microorganism brought a schism to the clinic, between the disease and the patient, between the patient and the remedy and between the different parts of the organism itself.

The idea of the organism fighting the poison and the remedy fighting the cause corresponds to the separation between the patient, the disease and the prescription. The remedy became specific to each disease and no longer to the patient, and more: specific to the cause of the disease, not to its consequences in the body. The absence of an etiologic agent definitively created the specific disease. And this creation oriented all other medical disciplines - including physiopathology - towards the identification of specific diseases, individualized by their etiologies.

Etiological reasoning characterizes the disease to be combated as something eliminable, foreign, causing limited disorders and, it should be noted, specific to each disease and not to each patient. In this way, medicine consolidated its current conceptions and, above all, its precise objectives: to cure and prevent diseases as a method of treating the sick. From then on, proposals for individualized treatment of pathophysiological disorders no longer made sense. These methods ultimately focused on the whole organism, the body, which was understood to be dysfunctional or unbalanced.

The proposals of therapists, who until the 19th century sought to understand functional disorders in the body as arising from its own dynamism, fighting the idea of disease as a specific being, were defeated. Microbiology gave illness an autonomous existence, showed itself on the empirical terrain of the microscope, and gave it an uncomfortable consistency.

But until Pasteur, criticism of the use of medicines was more focused on finding effective remedies for the individual patient. With the advent of microbiology, medical dreams of a therapy centered on the patient and the recovery of their health were overtaken. Pasteur also gave birth to another branch of microbiology, Hygiene. Not Hygiene, health through PHYSIS, but Hygiene - the prevention of disease.

The 19th century doctor followed the path of the Enlightenment and maintained his medicine on the basis of a beneficial nature. Microbiology transforms this action. Contemporary science does not listen to nature in order to heal itself, because it does not attribute positive value to it; it seeks to dominate it and subject it to its own designs, of which healing can be a part. This cure is not, however, a process of improvement, as the Greeks wanted with Hygeia, nor is it transformative, of mutation brought about by external forces, as Panacea would be. This is because the disease was caused by external nature and the cure is the result of the struggle that follows the invasion of man by elements of this alien environment.

This dilution of the uniqueness of each human being contributes to the loss of the notion of individual health, a state of excellence proper to each being, to be replaced by the idea of "normal". For contemporary medicine, the ideas of health or cure are replaced by those of normal or return to normal, and this normality ultimately means the absence of disease or the end of disease.

By placing disease in the environment and giving it an ontological status, contemporary medicine removes the discussion of health from the properly human terrain. In addition, the expansion of hygiene tools won over public authorities, government elites and all those who dreamed of a more regulated society free from epidemics. This conception created a new medical myth: that each professional would be a guardian of society in the fight to extinguish disease, rather than a therapist. The figure of the therapist is then weakened and loses importance. Because the myth of science to extinguish diseases turns him into a disciplinarian, a purveyor of preventive and healthy rules and behaviours, organized to control both external nature and human nature.

In this way, the doctor-patient relationship ceases to exist as a space for interpersonal exchanges, because it is codified by the medical order: the doctor doesn't need to care for the patient, just control their illness, rationalize and discipline their fears and teach them to be obedient to the rules of good conduct.

On the other hand, countless links can be made between scientific rationality and social organization, and at any given time many individual factors in the private sphere escape the standardized application of more or less technical principles. Therapeutic activity, among others, can either be entirely subject to the dictates of the medical order or entirely escape its norms.

It can be a wish or a dream for a cure, whether it comes from the heart of the patient or the therapist, whether they are Hippocratic or Mezzo-scientist, expectant or interventionist. The biggest problem for today's doctor is seeing the unique phenomenon of each living being in a synthetic, total way. This is because healing is, in essence, the result of a process of relationship between the patient and the world, the doctor and his prescription.

The doctor exists to mediate the encounters capable of producing the changes necessary for healing in the patient's life. And healing capacity is not, in turn, related to a cognitive parameter, but rather to an unmeasurable and timeless expectation: the end of suffering and incapacity and, ultimately, the desire to live and stay away from death.

Medicine, like other activities, is confused at the moment, convinced that it must become a science in terms of rigor and precision. This is a difficult situation, because the doctor, master of the secrets of his art, is a wise double of an artist, in other words, the embodiment of the highest and most complete intelligence. In the words of Fonsagrives (a 19th century French doctor): "Let us be scientific artists, but let us remain artists".

For this author, the notion of medicine as art as opposed to science is not to be confused with the old argument between science and practice, which is actually a false question. It is not a question of understanding art as the practical application of a theoretical science; the main aspect of art is its synthetic nature and the fact that it requires sensitivity to the specificities of each situation in which it is applied. This art of medicine is all about therapeutics, its ultimate goal and the source of all the dignity of its exercise.

Sayd's (1998) historical approach shows an idealized medical practice when focused on therapeutics. She also recognizes that the use of a scientifically valuable arsenal of drug therapies is very recent and insufficient for a broader approach to the demands of patients' suffering. The author therefore emphasizes the doctor's ability to mediate and remedy, in other words, to apply other therapeutic modalities, historically consecrated, not only for their technique, but also for their value in the art of healing.

Based on Sayd's (1998) elaboration, we will consider the possibility of reframing acupuncture therapy through the prism of remediation.

9 Therapeutics: The world of medicines

According to the Education Portal (2016), a remedy can be defined by its ability to cure. It can be an animal, vegetable, mineral or synthetic substance. It can be a procedure such as gymnastics, massage, baths or acupuncture. It can be faith or belief, used with beneficial intent.

Nowadays, based on the medical rationality seen above, we can easily understand why the scientific literature on remedies has been replaced by that on medicines. The same portal defines a medicine as a drug with scientifically proven beneficial properties. So let's again turn to the experience of the acupuncture apprentice to try to elucidate why the education portal defines acupuncture as a medicine.

Nightmares and pain:

The patient was accompanied by a diagnosis of hypothyroidism due to Hashimoto's thyroiditis. She had an enlarged gland and an ultrasound showing a heterogeneous pattern with micronodules. The patient had a small rise in her thyroid-stimulating hormone, with no other symptoms. She was a late puerpera, but no longer breastfed her son. She believed she was going through a difficult phase, trying to reconcile her professional and married life with the new birth. She seemed frustrated and tired at times and complained of not having enough time for herself. The patient began to suffer from repetitive nightmares with content

of worry about her son, accompanied by body movements during the night. She got up and walked around the house in her sleep and one night she fell to the floor, cracking her right shoulder.
She was referred to acupuncture on the understanding that this therapeutic

modality could benefit her twice over: relieving her nightmares and easing the pain resulting from the shoulder trauma.

The patient was given explanations of the benefits of acupuncture based on Traditional Chinese Medicine knowledge, as well as those derived from biomedical knowledge about acupuncture's mechanisms of action on pain.

The patient underwent needling by a professional qualified in both approaches. She reported a feeling of slight pain when the needles were inserted, pressure on some points and temporary burning. This was followed by a sensation of deepening of her breathing and a feeling of generalized muscle relaxation, especially a feeling of lightness in her head. The patient reported that, at the end of the sessions, her feeling was one of general well-being and that, during the breaks in her routine, she noticed an increase in her physical disposition, relief from the pain in her right shoulder and a significant improvement in her mood, although this was not a complaint prior to the acupuncture sessions. The nightmares stopped completely.

Regardless of the interpretations derived from the knowledge about the efficacy of acupuncture, we observed the description of a therapeutic phenomenon, that is, a practice of inserting needles into specific points of a suffering body, which resulted in an increase in its vitality and an improvement in its quality of life, together with the relief of complaints prior to the establishment of the therapy: nightmares and pain.

10 Acupuncture from the Vitalist Paradigm

In her article: A formação medica sob a otica do paradigma vitalista: via de entrada em um novo mundo, Maria Ines Nogueira (2013) states that since primitive civilizations (Assyrian-Babylonian, Egyptian, Iranian) there would have been a "vitalist paradigm" and that it would have crossed Indian and Chinese cultures, persisting in ancient Greece and Rome and influencing the Medical Schools of Antiquity.

From this thought arises the power of each being to reconstitute itself, or to remain whole, in a relationship of harmony in coexistence with other living beings, where nature is a shaper, maintainer and healer. This ideal was present in Hippocratic medicine and persisted until the 19th century. With the emergence of anatomoclinical medicine, another style of thought was consolidated, where disease was no longer a vital phenomenon, but an expression of tissue and cell damage. The disease-injury diary became the central category of medical knowledge and practice. Despite the importance of this Hippocratic model, it lacked a well-structured therapeutic system.

Despite the hegemony of biomedicine, in the 20th century, from the 1960s onwards, there was a revival of the vitalist perspective in the area of health, driven by the counter-culture movement. With the impact of these ideas on Western society, later disseminated by the World Health Organization (WHO), there was a growing rise of all rationalities and practices that share a vitalist perspective.

It is therefore possible to see the coexistence of two health paradigms in today's medicine: the vitalist and the biomedical. These are the paradigms that underpin the different complex medical systems or "Rationalities".

Medical"

The Biomedical Paradigm, built on the objectification of health problems, allows for the control of the biological and social body. The Vitalist Paradigm values the subjective dimensions present in illness, favoring disease prevention, health promotion and comprehensive care. This line of reasoning considers that all medical education is conditioned by a Paradigm or a Style of Thought and occurs through examples and manuals with an emphasis on training, exercises and repetition. The author concludes her text by explaining that the education process can be understood as training with the aim of transmitting not only cognitive content, but also a different way of defining what "reality" is.

Thus, if we consider the need for a differentiated training process, the introduction of new practice scenarios in medical training is intended to critically reorient the learner's gaze: from an anatomical gaze to an expanded one. Entering a new world, with different ways of seeing, speaking, writing and acting.

Returning to the clinical case of the patient with pain and nightmares, I believe we can say that acupuncture worked as a remedy for this patient and, consequently, her acupunctured body became a "remedied body". But in order to understand how this "remedied body" is constituted, we have to make another concept of intelligibility of this body available: the concept of "embodiment".

11 Embodiment" in Acupuncture

In the biomedical model, the body is defined in a relatively stable, predictable way, as an objective entity. It is understood as a complex biochemical machine that can be repaired by medical intervention (Freund and Macguire, 1999). Disease in this model is understood to be caused by a specific, identifiable agent, and the body in this model is a self-evident body (Howson, 2013).

The importance of this mechanistic concept of the body is to understand its relative shielding, which presupposes a therapeutic medical intervention based on the same understanding, i.e. the poor understanding of the environment's relationship with this body and the predictability of the body's responses in relation to its interactions with the environment. This environment, in turn, is broadly made up of the socio-economic-cultural and psychic-emotional environments.

In contrast to this model of the body that excludes itself from relationships with its environment, Flores-Pereira (2010) presents another understanding of the body, the person body *(embodiment),* which sees the body as more than a representational object, seeking to understand it as a constitutive part of the person, an agent capable of building the history and culture of the space where it lives.

The author draws on the theories of Csordas (1994) and Merleau-Ponty (2001) to show the possibility of the body as more than a biological object, moving on to an understanding of the body as social and an important actor in the construction of society. From its ability to see, hear, smell, taste, speak, feel, touch, explore and desire, in other words, from phenomenological experience, the body constitutes the person in relation to the world.

Flores-Pereira (2010) informs *us* that *"embodiment"* is the nomenclature that has been primarily used to talk about this fundamental and intertwined relationship that is created between the body and the socio-historical-cultural world. This experience, for Flores-Pereira (2010), is that of the body-person, experiencing a world of practice and not of abstraction.

If we interpret the body as a relational body, the theory of *"embodiment"* seems more realistic for analyzing what we observe in the practice of acupuncture. According to Howson (2013), *"embodiment"* can be used in different ways, but it is usually done from two aspects, both of which emphasize the interrelationships between biological and social processes. The concept can therefore be used to emphasize the body as a living instance of human experience, as well as alerting us to the relationship between the object, external and institutionalized body and the sensitive, subjective body.

Another aspect of the concept of "*embodiment*" is the affirmation of bodily integrity as the center of self-identity, which can be observed in practices that take place through bodily work. This bodywork can come from the body as an agent, which responds to and creates the social world through the senses and meanings attributed to action and bodily practices, or from the body as "*embodiment*" itself, where the body is confused with the concept of self-embodiment, or as we saw earlier, the body-person of Flores-Pereira (2010).

In this way, the concept of *"embodiment"* presupposes an understanding of the body based on practice, affirming that the body's relationship with the environment is one of incorporation, constituting its identity as an incorporated self.

In the case of acupuncture as a body or body-localized practice, we can apply the concept of *"embodiment"* to allude to the body that incorporates this therapeutic environment, which includes the application of needles at specific points on the body, and in turn the body remedies and the needles remedy the suffering represented or identified in the incorporated self, constituting this body as the "remedied body".

Therefore, to look at the "remedied body" is to observe a product of acupuncture practice and at the same time the possibility of understanding the *"embodiment"* of this body, in other words, the environmental or biopsychosocial conditions that constituted it as a self-embodiment of suffering.

Another example that can make this perspective clearer can be found in the book Trigger Point Treatment: A Guide to Pain Management by Clair and Amber Davis (2012). In the chapter where the authors teach massage therapists how to treat trigger points, they also state that the logic behind the technique of massaging myofascial anatomical structures, which are recognized as causing pain, is that the therapist should only create conditions that promote healing, as it would be foolish to think that therapists have a significant degree of direct control over the body. The therapist should, however, stimulate the healing process that is carried out by the body itself.

The authors also state that it would be counterproductive to over-treat, as we must trust the body. Furthermore, in agreement with Travell (1992), everyone's body is different to some degree, requiring carefully differentiated and specific treatment. They emphasize that we should not rely on protocols but on the patient as our best teacher.

Although Davis (2012) understands that it is important to know the detailed anatomical structure that allows us to understand the location of the trigger points to be treated, they employ vitalist cosmology, understanding that it is this body that is remedied, from the neurophysiological stimulus used in an individualized way and from the "*embodiment*" of a world of relationships that constitutes each embodied self of pain.

12 Final considerations:

In this paper, we tried to answer the question of which body is subjected to acupuncture. The conclusion of the "remedied body" was built on the understanding that both styles of thought, traditional and Western, justify the efficacy of acupuncture, i.e. its therapeutic effect, but do not explain the phenomenon of acupuncture itself.

This is why we used the concept of *"embodiment"* to point out that, regardless of the assumptions from which the acupuncture apprentice explains the benefits of this practice to his patient and his peers, it is the "body remedied" by acupuncture, as a phenomenon produced by this practice, that guarantees its permanence as an established therapy in the East and West, because it is characterized by a therapeutic body practice to remedy a self-embodied suffering.

Therefore, we end with the possibility of understanding that acupuncture's mechanisms of action and Chinese patterns of disharmony are more important for the legitimacy of the practice of acupuncture, because it is based on knowledge-power, a Foucauldian concept, than for understanding the phenomenon of this practice.

I believe we can conclude, in the approach of this work, that the possibility of observing the appearance of the "body remedied" by acupuncture, based on the phenomenon of *"embodiment"*, explains both its effectiveness and its stability sufficiently.

Bibliographical references:

Campbell, A. (2001) Acupuncture in practice: beyond points and meridians. Butterworth-Heinemann, Edinburgh.

Csordas, T. Emdodiment and Experience. Cambridge: Cambridge University Press, 1994.

Davies. C. Trigger Point Therapeutic Book: pain treatment guide. Sao Paulo: Roca, 2012.

Douglas, M. Natural Symbols: Explorations in Cosmology. New York: Pantheon, 1970.

FLORES-PEREIRA, Maria Tereza. **Body, person and organizations.** *Organ. Soc.* [online]. 2010, vol.17, n.54, pp. 417-438. ISSN 1984-9230.

FREUND, P; MCGUIRE, M. Illness and the Social Body. Upper Saddle River, New Jersey: Prentice Hall, 1999.

Foucault, M. As palavras e as coisas: uma arqueologia das ciencias humanas. Sao Paulo: Martins Fontes, 1987, p. 407 p.

HACKING, I. *The social construction of what?* Cambridge, Massachusetts and London, England: Harward University Press, 1999.

HOWSON. A. The body in society: An introduction. Cambridge: Polity Press, 2013.

Kaptchuk T.J. (1983) Chinese Medicine: the web that has no weaver. Hutchinson Publishing Group, London.

KLEINMAN, A. *The illness narratives:* Basic Books, 1988.

KRUSE, M. H.L, Anatomy: the order of the body. *Rev Bras Enferm,* Brasilia (DF) 2004 jan/feb;57(1):79-84.

Kuriyama S. (2000) The Expressiveness of the Body and the Divergence of Greek and Chinese Medicine. Zone Books, New York.

Levi-Strauss, C. O Pensamento Selvagem. Sao Paulo: Ed. Nacional, 1976, p.331.

Merleau-Ponty, M. Phenomenology of Perception. London: Routledge, 2001.

NEI CHING: *The Golden Book of Chinese Medicine.* Second edition. Rio de Janeiro: EDITORA OBJETIVA LTDA. 165p.

Nogueira, M. I.

SANTOS, B. S. *The critique of indolent reason: against the waste of experience.* Sao Paulo: Cortez, 2005.

SAYD, J. *Mediar, Medicar, Remediar:* aspectos da terapeutica na Medicina Ocidental. Rio de Janeiro: EdUERJ, 1998.

Travell, J. G; Simons, D. G. Myofascial Pain and Dysfunction: The Trigger Point Manual. Baltimore: Lippincott, 1992.

TURNER, B. S. Regulating Bodies: Essays in Medical Sociology. London: Sage, 1992.

Education Portal:
http://www.portaleducacao.com.br/enfermagem/artigos/681/farmacologia-conceitos-basicos#ixzz41JBgpIp9. Accessed on 28/02/2016.

Index

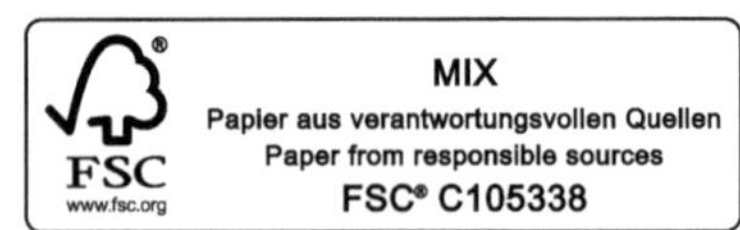

Printed by Books on Demand GmbH, Norderstedt / Germany